I Love Life

To my Son

Golin'

Love

Mum

Also by Dorthy Calcutt

The Salt of the Earth (1999)
Born in a Stable (2001)
My Three Hats (2003)

I Love Life

The NHS is ours: let's take care of it

Dorothy Calcutt

THE WYCHWOOD PRESS

Our books may be ordered from bookshops or (post free) from
The Wychwood Press, Alder House, Market Street, Charlbury, OX7 3PH
01608 811969

e-mail: wychwood@joncarpenter.co.uk

Credit card orders should be phoned or faxed to 01689 870437 or 01608 811969

Please send for our free catalogue

First published in 2004 by
The Wychwood Press
an imprint of Jon Carpenter Publishing
Alder House, Market Street, Charlbury, Oxfordshire OX7 3PH

ISBN 1 902279 19 0

Printed in England by Antony Rowe Ltd., Eastbourne

Contents

1	As we were	8
2	Struggling	10
3	From Wingfield to Nuffield	13
4	From war to peace	15
5	Moulding together	18
6	Individual attention	21
7	Into the N.H.S.	24
8	The build-up	26
9	Out of this world	29
10	Take up thy bed and walk	32
11	Witney Community Hospital	35
12	A night on the tiles	39
13	Home again	43
14	Looking forward with hope	47

Acknowledgements

I would like to thank my daughter Madge, who has put this book on computer. Also my son in law Richard who took and developed the photographs. To Bridget who jotted notes for me when my state of health was tottering. To both Madge and Bridget for more photographs.

Also to everyone else, family or village friends – far too numerous to mention by name.

To all the staff in all the hospitals and my own general practitioner. Working together we have conquered.

Preface

I was born in 1920, received no medical attention at birth. I suffered from all the children's illnesses but no doctor was ever called.

I was taken to the local practitioner in 1927 with a broken arm. That cost my parents seven shillings and sixpence, the price of a farm worker's weekly wage at the time.

Because we paid a hospital weekly subscription, I was allowed into the maternity unit for my first baby in 1946.

My second baby, born in 1947, I had at home and needed to pay for visits by the district nurse and doctor. The hospital did not cater for any babies after the first.

Now we are fully catered for, yet people grumble about it and badly abuse it.

Let's take care of ourselves and each other; the hospitals get filled with many that smoke, or are too fat, drink too much alcohol or are careless road users.

There are enough illnesses without self-inflicted ones. I hope you enjoy this book and contribute in one small way to improving the situation.

Dorothy Calcutt

1 As we were

For hundreds of years scholars have marvelled at the miracle of the human body, but not until the sixteenth century did William Harvey fathom the circulation of the blood. It was about the same time that ether was discovered, but it was years later when it was first used as an anaesthetic.

Queen Victoria who had so many children but, hating the pain that was involved, decided that she must be given ether to ease that pain. It was her own son; Edward seventh whose coronation was postponed because he had a successful appendix operation. Surgery has multiplied since then but it is only about one hundred years old.

Building the Radcliffe Infirmary began about seventeen seventy and was used mostly for patients who were close to death and in so much pain it was impossible for them be kept at home. Most families – some very large – lived in two bedroom cottages. Often they housed a grandparent, when one was ill it was difficult to manage. The bedroom contained small children, the patient and a much needed commode. Lavender was kept smouldering to ease nature's smells, that were abundant. Very few poor children attended school, why should they? They only needed to learn things that would help towards a livelihood. So most girls were directed towards private service when they were about ten years old. This was done partly to help the girls but mostly to relieve the overcrowding at home. The mistress of the new house undertook the upbringing of the girl from that time.

It was during these years that the Girl's Friendly Society started, because so many of these girls were getting into trouble or running away. The G.F.S was held on one evening each week and the girls had about two hours for recreation. Sometimes they listened to a talk about good housekeeping:-

How to light a fire,
How to clean and fill a paraffin lamp,
How to peel vegetables very thinly,
How to sharpen a knife.

These were the real basics, that would stand them in good stead when they finally married.

If they attended the meetings for three whole years they would be presented with a certificate by one of the employers. I still have one of my mothers, that she had framed in 1910 when she was sixteen.

Boys were always kept at home to encourage work and pay something into the family kitty.

In 1876 my great uncle John was taken ill. Although illegitimate, his father was rich and had always provided for him. He took him in his own carriage to the Radcliffe Infirmary, only to be told that he would most likely die. It was meningitis, but Mr Henry Acland did all he could, helping other would-be doctors as he did so. This was a good source of money.

All John's friends that he had left behind said that the illness was caused by too much education; his brain had been overworked and caused the illness. He did recover but that 'old wives tale' continued until quite recent years.

This work at the Infirmary by Mr Acland and his colleagues helped the progress of medicine.

The next time I heard of doctors helping my family was in November 1918. My father plus three other members of the same chapel all suffered from Spanish flu. His cousin, Lora Walker and a Mr Oldacre both died but Miss E. Putt – the organist – and my father recovered.

That boxing day my father cycled to Woodstock to call a doctor to the birth of their first baby. Dr Mogg got out his motorbike and said he would be coming through the park. However the snow was too deep, so he was obliged to leave his bike in a drift and walk on.

2 Struggling

The Radcliffe Infirmary now needed financial support, so all the villages in the catchment area were asked to collect 2d a week from all married couples and 1d a week from all over fourteen. My father offered to collect in one part of Combe. This was a job for my sister and me each Friday. At the end of the quarter all the collectors in Combe took their money to dad, he counted it and sent it in by the courier. At Easter we made a special collection of eggs. Most cottagers kept hens and they always laid well in the spring but stopped as the days got shorter. This ensured that each patient had a boiled egg for Easter Sunday breakfast.

The Infirmary had expanded in size. There were two large wards for males and two for females. Matrons began to discipline the nurses and the air was now filled with carbolic and lysol.

Sir Henry Acland had already established a link between hospital and university. New ideas and remedies were tried on very willing recipients whose days were already numbered.

Most families lived in such close proximity that children's complaints multiplied and the infant death rate was very, very high. Any premature baby or weakling stood very little chance of living.

Workhouses were being used for families who could not find work. Many jobs included a tied cottage and often these situations resulted in the family being thrown onto the street. I myself remember it happening. The hours that were worked or the price per hour that labourers received was never monitored. A workman was a commodity, not a human being with feelings.

Small towns had set up homes in isolated places for those with infectious diseases. They were often called 'pest houses' and the inhabitants were treated as scum, blackguards or scoundrels. They were in fact very unlucky individuals who had met both with dreadful complaints and unforgiving employers. Poverty controlled both life and family and it carried through from generation to generation.

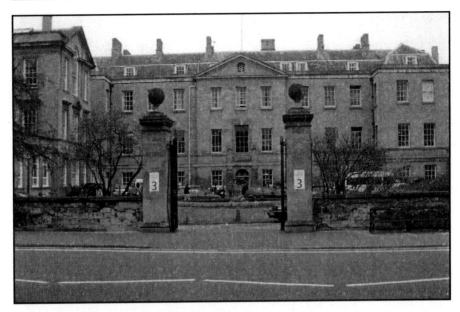

Above: The entrance to the Radcliffe Infirmary.

Below: The eye hospital adjacent to the Radcliffe Infirmary.

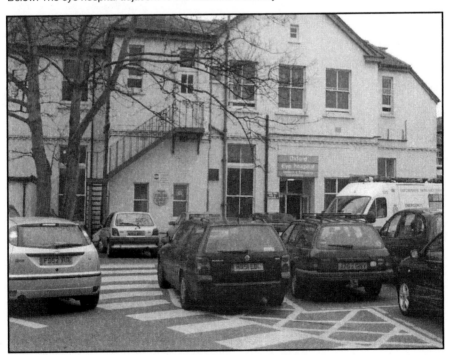

People did not suffer quite so badly in areas of industry. The coal mines, the iron and steel industries and the textile factories were all a blessing but in rural areas the only employers were connected with the land. A man would boast that he was a ploughman, a milkman or a gamekeeper. Whatever he was he had to be content with the lowest wage. (Very few women went out to work but they often took in jobs that could be done at home. In our area that was gloving.)

Farm workers were always looked down upon. Their education was limited as was their mobility. Their life style was physically hard but plenty of fresh air ensured that they did not suffer from chest infections, as did the miners. During these years the Infirmary developed both a maternity ward and a separate section for the study of eye weaknesses.

3 From Wingfield to Nuffield

About one hundred years after the building of the Radcliffe Infirmary, Mrs Wingfield decided that a convalescent home should be built to help patients recover from illnesses.

She built a hospital – The Wingfield – for this purpose. This ensured that recovery was given a special place. There were very few operations at this time, and no antibiotics or plaster. They were using splints for broken bones but money was very scarce so most of the working class who managed to break a bone ... too bad, they were left untreated.

Oxford was considered a rich town, housing so many from the university. They could afford such lavish treatment.

The Wingfield developed over the years into a special hospital for infectious illnesses that needed patients to be isolated. In the 1920s it was used for tuberculosis and poliomyelitis. We all used solid fuel fires and smoke was prevalent in cities, producing very bad fogs which even then were considered to be dangerous to the

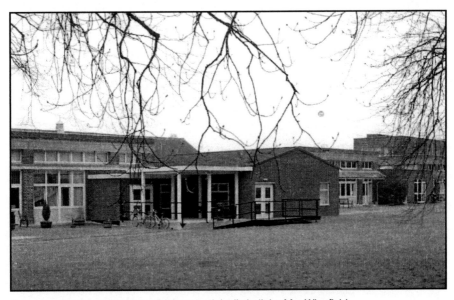

A panoramic view of the Noc, which was originally built by Mrs Wingfield.

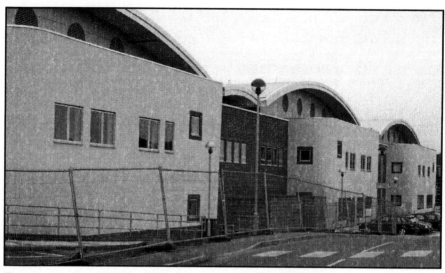

The new part of the Nuffield, nearly ready to welcome its first patients.

lungs. For this reason this hospital was built on the outskirts of the town.

Mr William Morris bought two iron lungs for polio victims at a cost of one million pounds each. That was an awful lot of money but travel was getting easier, so people were needing to use the facilities. Morris was now selling lots of cars, making more work for the locals, more money for himself, and those very cars he produced were beginning to cause accidents and filled that hospital.

He put millions of pounds into that side of medicine. When he was given the title of Lord Nuffield, the name of the hospital was changed to the Nuffield Orthopaedic Centre. It was devoted solely to that purpose. Those connected with it now quite lovingly refer to it as 'The Noc'.

Two benefactors had produced this specialist hospital very near to the foot of Shotover.

4 From war to peace

During the Second World War the Americans needed somewhere for soldiers who were wounded in action. It had to be in the south of England and not too far from Brize Norton aerodrome. They chose a spot not far from the Nuffield and where the population was sparse to avoid the chance of bombing. It was constructed very quickly but served its purpose well. They called it 'The Churchill' and when the Americans moved out at the end of the war it was used for a myriad of complaints. I've known it to be used for maternity, one-day operations, chest complaints and cancer.

Oxford could not manage without this facility. This was now the third hospital that Oxford had received without money from the government. The population was expanding rapidly, the number of complaints that could be treated and cured was rising.

Is progress always beneficial? It was at this time that cars began to overtake the need for trains. The domination of cars produced far more accidents than trains. Those same cars that gave us so

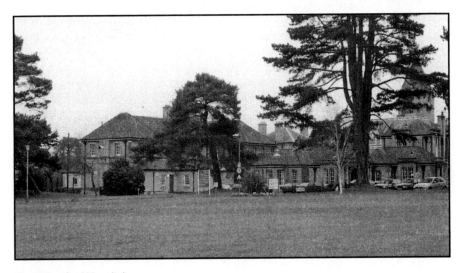

The Warneford Hospital.

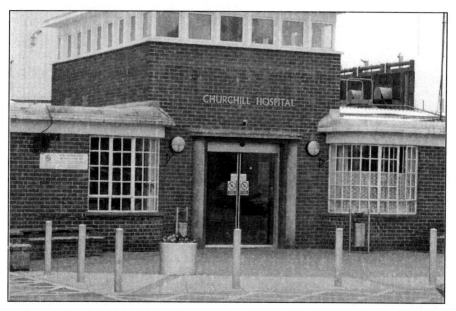

Above: The main entrance to the original Churchill Hospital.
Below: The entrance to the most recent part.

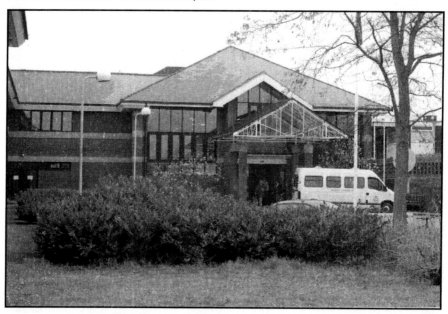

many jobs also filled our hospitals.

Since the Churchill was built it has been modernised and refurbished several times. It now treats many forms of cancer, chest and skin complaints. Infectious diseases are also catered for.

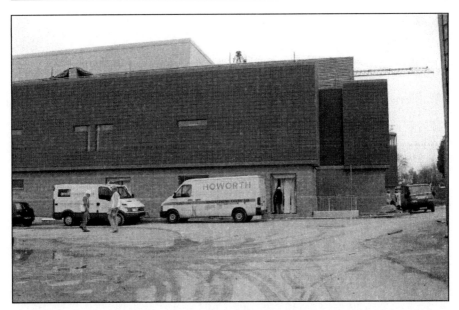

The new Acland Hospital: a private building to replace the Acland Home in Banbury Road.

At this time and for many years earlier a home at Littlemore catered for those with mental problems. The only mental hospital in Oxford now is the Warneford, smaller and not far from the Noc and the Churchill.

Even at the turn of the twentieth century a Dr Acland had started his private home in the Banbury Road for those who could afford it. In 2003 his successors started work on a new home in Headington. This will still be used by those of us who can afford it or those who fancy that individual attention.

Health facilities were expanding while the need for such valuable assets was ever increasing. More operations, more X-rays, more drugs, more asthma, more diabetes were all demanding more hospitals.

5 Moulding together

The government decided in the early seventies that one large encompassing hospital should be built. This was going to be the best ever, and it would cater for maternity and accident and emergency among all the other ailments. The maternity unit should open first. A beautiful building was built on the slopes of Headington. It can be seen for miles, the envy of all those around. Although it now caters for many hundreds and thousands, so far no other hospital has been closed.

This, The John Radcliffe, has proved to be an extra for every illness. The eye hospital has been left abutting the old Infirmary. Brain operations are still carried out there as well. The J.R. now stands proudly welcoming all who need its protection, smiling down on all the expectant users in the area. I would think that that square mile around Headington boasts more hospitals than anywhere else in the world.

Perhaps 'The Noc' would not be needed? No way! A hugh annexe has been built there to open in 2004, to be used among

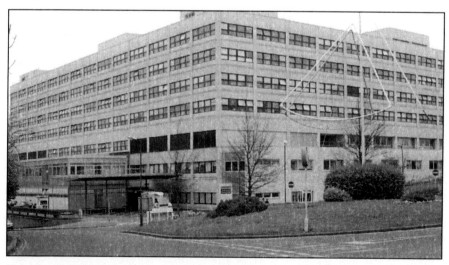

The John Radcliffe smiles down on the dreaming spires.

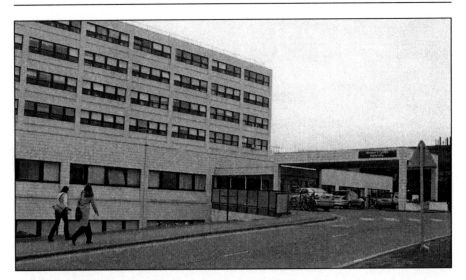

The Women's Hospital at the JR.

other things for research and teaching. It was badly needed, but our way of life in the twenty-first century is proving to be very harmful to our bodies. Pollution from cars, eating too much of the wrong food, drinking and smoking too much, too little exercise all manage to fill every available bed. (Very small families that have been reared in an affluent society have produced many selfish individuals. This is easily seen on the roads. If we all travelled within the stipulated speed limit we would not need humps in the road or traffic restrictions. If we all took responsibility to dispose of our own litter, there would be none blowing about in our hedgerows. I don't throw it there, you don't throw it there, but someone does.)

And even as I write a huge children's hospital is already under construction near the J.R. It will be unequalled in catering for the children.

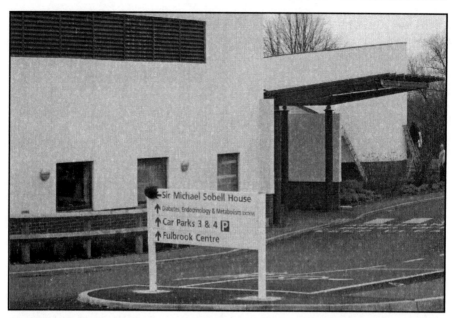

Sir Michael Sobell House (above) caters for terminal cancer patients over 40, while Helen House (below) caters for those under 18 who need long-term care.

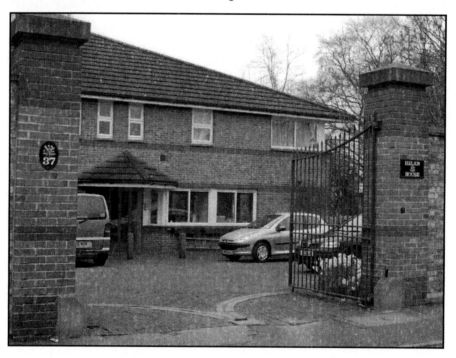

6 Individual attention

Elsewhere in Oxford the Rivermead Hospital caters for those who have suffered strokes and need much physiotherapy.

A home has been built near the Churchill and named Sobell House. It is used for cancer patients who need lots of attention but have little chance of being cured.

We then hear of Sister Frances who thought that children with these same problems should be housed separately. With her determination Helen House was built so as to be multipurpose, a functional yet beneficial home for the youngest members of society who have such a sad start in life.

Many of these youngsters have no chance of pursuing a good quality of life, but, as they grow older they need as much normal living as they can individually handle. What a consolation and relief, too, for the parents and other siblings left behind! When these afflicted members of the family live together, the rest of the family can suffer.

With this in mind Sister Frances and her helpers have now designed The Douglas House for those between eighteen and forty. It has recently been opened by the Queen. Residents have a games room, a music room, a swimming pool and a bar, as well as a corridor wide enough to race wheelchairs. Many other facilities are provided making it the best and possibly the only place of its kind in the world. It is the most homely, convenient and near luxurious surroundings they could possibly live in.

Many of the smaller towns in the surrounding area have their own community hospital where your own general practitioner oversees your well-being. They take those from the area who, say, have had a fall and need a few days of help and those who have come from intensive care and need a longer time to rehabilitate before going home.

Each town or large village has its own team of doctors and nurses. They listen to your symptoms and issue tablets of every

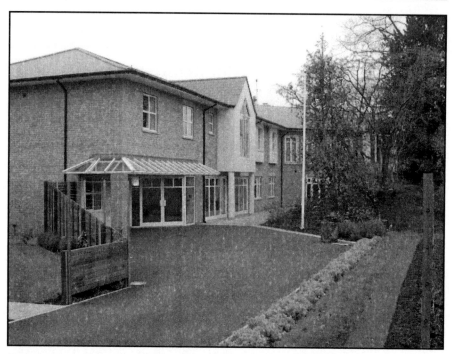

Douglas House caters for long-term patients aged between 18 and 40.

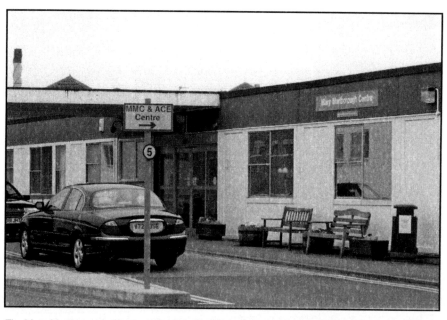

The Mary Marlborough Centre at the Noc finds occupational aids for patients recently released from the hospital.

sort. The nurses do pre-natal work, give injections, bandage sores and take blood samples. Each member of the team is very necessary; without any one of them this carefully designed system would begin to panic and shudder.

Wheels only work smoothly if each cog is straight and reliable. The health service is exactly the same. All teams are built on co-operation and the health service is the biggest team in the country.

To supplement this interlaced and complex system of health centres, small convalescent homes, both private and state, have sprung up to address each individual need. Carers will call daily and many accessories are lent according to your needs. There is a department of The Noc that shows you all the aids that are available for the disabled.

7 Into the N.H.S.

I started my family in 1946 but as this was my first baby I was taken into the maternity unit at the Radcliffe Infirmary for free. It would allow first babies to be catered for, but no others who had no complications. There was no charge while I was in the hospital but outside I paid for everything I needed. My second baby, born in 1947, was rather expensive. I had to pay for every visit by the district nurse. At the birth I paid for 'gas and air' which I didn't use. The doctor was called so I had a bill from him as well.

This was soon after the end of the second world war. So many service personnel who had been starved of home life for several years were home again. They needed employment and houses and rightly deserved them.

Hadn't they given up years of their youth? Time cannot be recovered but these people demanded a house to settle in and a job to keep them afloat. Temporary prefabricated housing sprang up like mushrooms overnight; but such houses were welcomed. After such a national undertaking there was bound to be a baby boom.

It was in this situation that the government planned the National Health Scheme. Mr Aneurin Bevan worked on proposals that had been originally thought up by Lord Beveridge. They would start a scheme where each individual would be catered for from the cradle to the grave.

They manage even more than this now, as it all starts much earlier. They can help you even before conception.

This was the birth of the N.H.S. A scheme that has helped so many of us. We use it daily but it is often abused. It was started in July 1948. During its infancy the population found scores of sensible reasons to visit the doctor. Children's infections, coughs and colds, cuts and bruises all suggested a visit. None of these trivial complaints would ever have justified a visit beforehand. Our local unit had two doctors at the time and one nurse; now there are five doctors and probably twenty or more supporting staff.

But the population has multiplied and many more illnesses can be treated. Chronic complaints appear to be increasing. Diabetes raises its ugly head at any time, in both the young and the elderly. There are more ulcers and cancers and at the same time more can be done to help. The number of treatable complaints increases, research multiplies, and the way forward has no light at the end of the tunnel.

We can do very little to help, but have you got a conscience?

Do you drink too much alcohol?

Do you smoke?

Do you eat more than is good for you?

Are you a careless driver?

Do you take plenty of exercise?

Do you allow your child too many fast foods?

Many of us think that we have the human right to do exactly as we wish. This is true, but there are millions of us that have that identical human right and we all came into this world in the same way. Therefore, at birth everyone is equal. What we do with our lives is our own responsibility, who we listen to, who we respect or even who we insult all cultivate each individual character.

If you are reading this and the balance of your mind is sound, just take a card and write on it 'I LOVE LIFE'.

Place it in front of your car, or indeed at any appropriate point where you yourself feel that it is needed. If you are a landlord, put it on view in your bar. This is just to remind each one of us of our weaknesses and temptations.

Remember that the N.H.S. was born fifty-six years ago because the rank and file of our country had no access to medicine. Money ruled our health and life. Now we are all entitled to modern inventions, modern surgery – yet we still grumble about very small mishaps that we, as humans, always have.

8 The build-up

In 1957 my husband had much pain caused by his hips. He was then forty-seven years old and the pain had been building up for many years.

He was sent by our local doctor to the Nuffield. Mr. Scott was the consultant and he and others were facing this problem that seemed to be occurring more frequently. Hip replacements had not yet taken place.

They advised him to have a realignment of the left leg, just to see if it worked. They fractured the femur and put it in traction, then three weeks later he came home on crutches. After ten months he managed to return to work. He was doing a job that needed a lot of walking, so for several months I went with him.

It was clear to us then that he could not continue in that situation. Mr Scott often visited him to register his progress, but he was concerned, so he suggested a new operation that was being developed. This was the hip replacement that is done so successfully now.

This proved to be ideal; the pain was gone, although his leg was still at an angle that could never be altered, so he would never be able to ride a bicycle again. We managed to buy a small car with automatic gear change and he could go to work quite happily.

I was left at home with our four children and our large garden – at least the digging was left to me. I loved gardening and all four children were now at school. The eldest had already got to secondary school so money was very limited.

Within a few months Mr Scott had called him back to have his right hip replaced. He was extremely pleased as the other operation had been so successful. He could walk well now and our family worries appeared over for a while.

But the new material that had been used for the bone parts began to crumble and the decision was made to replace it with a tested and tried substitute. This meant that during the next few years he would have two more operations, but at the end of this and even to the end of his life his hips gave him no more trouble.

This is the way progressive medicine works; there must be pioneers who are willing to submit to trials, knowing they may or may not get the expected relief. If that operation proves successful, the patient has the satisfaction of knowing that many others will be relieved in years to come.

I continued in the garden, although my husband did the hoeing and weeding.

During the nineties my own hips were giving cause for concern. Had I been doing too much digging? We had both been brought up in very poor families. Was it possible that our diets were not balanced and perhaps the bones were affected?

It was decided in 1997 that I should have a right hip replacement. My husband was pleased that I should benefit from his efforts! He passed away that year before I had my operation.

I passed that goal post quite successfully knowing that as time progressed my left hip would receive the same treatment. In September 2002 I went for an X-ray, after which I was put on the waiting list; they assured me that it would be done in less than a year.

They confirmed what my own doctor had told me, that the pain was based wholly in my hip. My knee had been very painful. They said it was possible for me to have a local anaesthetic. I thought that was abhorrent, but, after pondering the point, I convinced myself that it was the best way forward for me. After a full anaesthetic I always suffered much sickness which lasted for weeks.

True to their word I received notice to report at the Nuffield on 28 July 2003. I was glad to get it over, especially when they rang me the following day and said 'Could I report a week earlier?' I arrived at the hospital on July 20 to have my operation the following day.

I underwent the usual interrogation, where they pointed out to me that they were not prepared to use a local anaesthetic. I accepted that and when asked about allergies I told them that my skin would not tolerate nylon. I knew they were now using nylon stockings for several days after the op. 'We do have some non-nylon stockings,' he said, so he put those on my feet before the op.

He seemed to think that was a trivial request. As all items are changed each day, when I became alert after the op I was already wearing nylon stockings.

Would it be too much to ask for a notice on my bed stating 'Use no nylon'? That would not cost much either in time or money. Other nurses did not know that non-nylon ones existed so I suffered unnecessarily.

This carried on until Thursday when the consultant said that my temperature was high. I casually mentioned that it always was high when I wore nylon. Off came the stockings but the damage had been done. The following day when the others who had had the identical operation were packing their clothes to go home, they came to me and said, 'We are sending you to the J.R. Their doctors are better equipped to look after you now.'

They did not even hint at what was causing such concern.

9 Out of this world

They neglected to tell me of my condition, or the cause, but at the J.R. there was a complete change. I was met at the entrance by doctors and nurses: pulling aside the oxygen mask, I asked them what exactly was wrong.

Even as I was being ushered into the building, the doctor at the head of my bed said: 'You have three things causing distress. You have a clot of blood on the lungs, your heart is beginning to grumble, and you have pneumonia. We are going to treat all three at once.' It was blunt, which was how I wanted it. I was then given one dose of heparin; it acts like warfarin, which then caused a haemorrhage in my wound.

During this period I was quite comfortable and in no pain: of course I had been given drugs. I did not feel that I was very ill.

I really must mention the nurses in the J.R. There were so many of all races and religions. They came from all over the world, they were efficient, understanding, pleasant and even homely. I think the petite Filipino nurses in their early twenties who had left their husbands and babies thousands of miles away were superb. They had been brought up to expect this sort of life. They were tough, tireless and tactful. They always faced you with a cheerful smile.

They loved to talk of their own country. I remember one individual who told me she was twenty-four and had left behind a husband and three babies. 'We were taught that the only alternative was poverty. Nursing was a class subject that was taught in school. I remember my first lesson on bedside manners,' she said. They speak so highly of Britain. 'We don't object to leaving our families because we know exactly what we are doing. Many return home when they have saved enough to buy a house. My husband is a chef, and when I have enough money he will bring the children and we will settle down together. He has many offers of work already,' she said expectantly.

She was sitting by my bed while I was drinking a boxed drink with a straw. She knew I had had very little to eat so she brought me this 'Ensure' which is a balanced meal. Whether she talked to keep my mind active or whether she loved her family and her country so much she never tired of talking about them, I do not know, but she conversed with me as if I was her best friend. The benefit we received from that chat was mutual.

I was allocated six units of blood, so she set up the drip. I was still in no pain but I felt very weak and sleepy, and completely exhausted.

I opened my eyes on hearing the voice of my own general practitioner, Dr Sally Hope.

'Oh, I am pleased to see you,' I said. 'But you will never believe where I've been.'

'Tell me,' she answered.

'You will only laugh,' I replied.

'Oh, no I won't. Try me,' she said.

'Well I have just been to heaven,' I said, thinking that she would think I had had a dream.

'Well, I'm not surprised, they have just resuscitated you. You had a cardiac arrest, but you are all right now.'

This was Sunday morning, when she wasn't even on duty and she had called to see me because she understood my situation.

Some of us complain about our doctors, don't we? Is she special? That familiar face appeared at the exact time when I needed her most. It was not her duty, she came as a friend, as indeed all of her patients are. Thank you, Sally.

I have two daughters. Madge, the elder, lives about fifty miles away, but she has retired from work, while Bridget – the younger – lives quite close but she is teaching and the summer holidays were just starting.

They carefully contacted each other to make sure that their visits did not coincide.

Bridget came in that evening and was called to see the doctor. He asked her if she knew my feelings about resuscitation. Bridget was shocked; she did not know that it had already happened once, so she answered in a positive way. 'My mum is as tough as old

Harry. She will pull through this,' she said emphatically.

She sat by my bed, wiped my brow with a damp flannel, fetched a few ice cubes and gave me a few sips of water.

She leaned over my bed, each of us consoling the other. 'Would you like me to stay tonight?' she whispered and I just nodded.

Madge arrived early next morning as Bridget went home to sleep.

It proved to be a very busy day, more units of blood, then they decided to insert a filter into my vein. They took me down to another level and inserted it into my groin, then when it was in the large vein that goes to the heart it was opened like an umbrella. This would prevent any blood clots reaching my heart. Although Madge could see what was happening on a monitor screen, I could not even feel it.

I merely felt very weak and extremely tired. I think that filter probably saved my life. Thank you very much to those who decided and carried out such an undertaking on such an old woman.

My temperature was starting to subside so I knew that I was conquering the pneumonia. The filter had taken care of the embolism but the operation incision was causing concern, as it was slow to heal and I could not be given warfarin. I received more blood so very, very gradually my strength was returning.

10 Take up thy bed and walk

I was being gently cared for by those marvellous nurses. Then, when washing my back, one said, 'You have a rash on your back.'

She called the doctor in to see it and he said immediately that it was caused by a certain antibiotic. Many doctors and nurses did not agree. 'It is caused by the bed linen. The actual starch and bleach the laundry uses is responsible for this.'

A heated discussion took place while Bridget listened. I think that was wrong, it should not have taken place in front of either her or me. This was obviously not a unique case, it had been causing trouble for years. I later heard of patients who took their own bed linen when entering the J.R.

The rash was dreadful, it spread over every bit of my body, ruined my nails and even weeks later I was still shedding my skin.

This should be sorted out. Could they be using some concoction to eliminate M.R.S.A., the superbug?

Is there a reason for starching sheets?

Is every hospital suffering?

I suffered with this for several weeks, and I do mean – *suffered*.

I have a family of four and they all supported me and I also live in a small village. Villagers are renowned for being busybodies and gossips. This is a myth that should be forgotten. When anything goes wrong they work as a unit and do everything possible; while patients around me were getting no visits, I always had visitors and my tables were full of flowers.

When you live in a small village you have a sense of belonging, it is like an extended family. I would like to thank each one of you; you automatically knew whether or not it was convenient to stay.

I was now only suffering from an operation scar, not yet healed, and a rash, so the J.R. said they were sending me back to the Noc. I also had a pain in the calf of my left leg, so I told them about it. They made no comment. Did they not hear me?

So I was moving bed again, the Foley Ward at the Noc was my

destination. As the paramedics wheeled me into the ambulance, one of them looked at me and said, 'Oh! Not you again!'

Any patient coming from a different hospital is taken to the Foley Ward. Tests were done to make doubly sure that I was not carrying that dreaded M.R.S.A. bug. After a few days there they decided to transfer me to the Mayfair Ward, in the private section.

They did not give me a reason. The rash was still distressing but the bed linen in those wards is blue – definitely not starched. This was my guess, they were spraying me frequently with calomine lotion. I am naturally a gregarious being, as indeed we all are. If we are alone we start complaining of loneliness. I would have preferred several patients in my ward, but there were only two beds and the other one was used for very short stay operations, usually just one day.

Apart from the coloured sheets there were very few differences. They did have thermos jugs for the water. That seemed a good idea, till I tried to pour some, only to find the jug was far too heavy so I could not lift it. That was sour grapes to me, and I was grateful for my frequent visitors again.

The food was extremely good, very little difference between the J.R. and the Noc. I did notice that when it was a fish day, in the J.R. we had cod, while in the Noc it was salmon. Once it was dover sole. I love cod and I often thought, what will happen when cod is more expensive than salmon? There is very little difference even now.

One of my daughters was usually there to help if I needed it at meal times. After a meal they would brush my dentures or cope with any small duties that arose.

I told the staff at the Noc about the pain in the calf of my left leg but like the J.R. they didn't even comment. Didn't they hear me either?

It was evident that after so many weeks in hospital, I would be sent to our community hospital in Witney. To be sent there was the first sign I was getting back to normal life. They would strive to get me walking again. My rash had not gone, but I had started to shed my skin. The rash was receding but the irritation was not.

So I was on the move again, much nearer to more familiar faces.

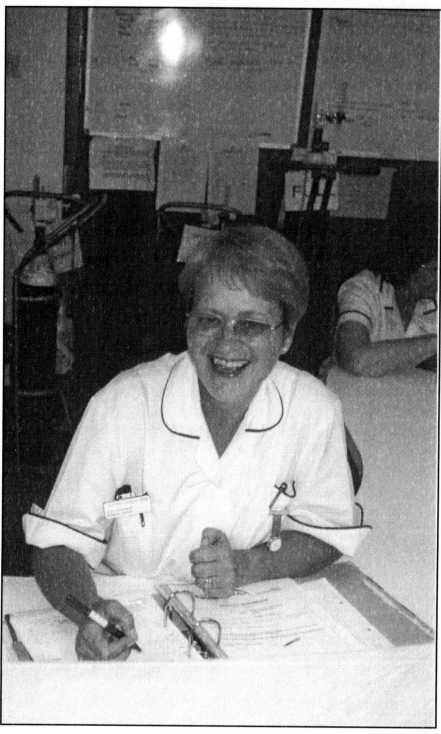

Liz at the controls in Witney Commnunity Hospital.

11 Witney Community Hospital

I spent many hours in Witney hospital just watching the skills of those nurses. Those noiseless, nifty beings that move in their own well-rehearsed corridor routine.

I wondered whether, when starting in the nursing profession, the first commandment is: Thou shalt not run.

The rhythm and flow of those nurses in those corridors is as recognisable as the square bashing of soldiers. I wonder if they use a tune to accomplish this feat. Certainly not 'Colonel Bogey'. They give the appearance of running a race, without trying to win. They all want to finish that race at precisely the same time, which is more difficult. As soon as they see a long corridor with daylight at the end, that corridor bounce surges up within them and away they go.

Sarah had perfected that bounce; she was young and nimble, and to add to this she had a long ponytail. This added to the bounce factor. Up and down the corridor all day long came the newly starched linen, the laundry basket, the drugs and meal trolleys, but nothing compared with the evening ritual.

Those of us that could get out of bed were given a commode at night, partly to prevent us from going to the toilet, waking others, maybe even falling or causing a commotion.

Several nurses brought those commodes down that same corridor. A traffic jam of commodes? Still the same bounce, together they came.

'Here we go, here we go, here we go.'

They didn't sing it, but I did, little did they realise what amusement they caused.

Witney is a friendly hospital, more like home, but it still has the motto, We will get you out of here as quickly as we can. Now we've all been cured. Or have we?

Physiotherapists worked on us all, walking aids were distributed, it was the patients' turn to work hard now while the nurses

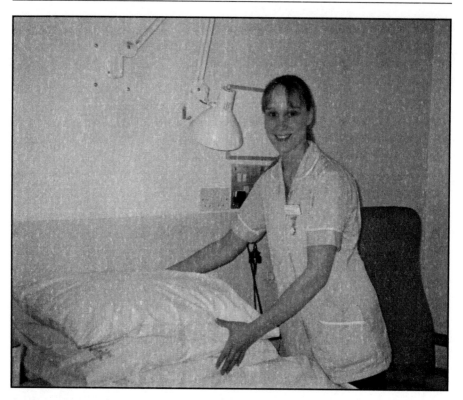

Sarah doing one of the many chores.

took care of us. The charge nurse was Liz. She was no old fashioned matron. She was disciplined and expected discipline, but very thorough.

I was there and was expected to walk but I could not. As soon as I started using a zimmer my left leg wouldn't move and I would collapse. The physio was persistent, and as I showed no improvement she concluded that I didn't really want to walk, or wasn't trying.

One morning when the ward was very quiet an unknown nurse came to see me. She explained that nurses were short on our ward so she had come from another ward. The nurses from our ward were having a discussion, she explained. 'I guess you don't know the topic,' she said, but I knew only too well they were talking about me.

This nurse took my perpetually monitored blood pressure, as I was lying on the bed. The she asked me to stand out of bed with

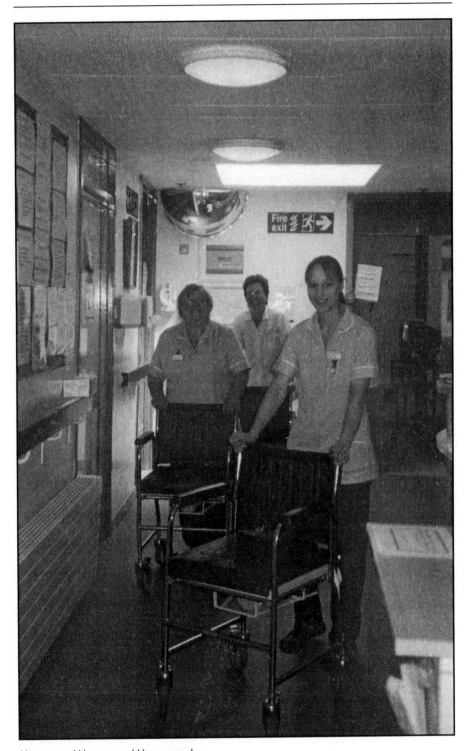

Here we go! Here we go! Here we go!

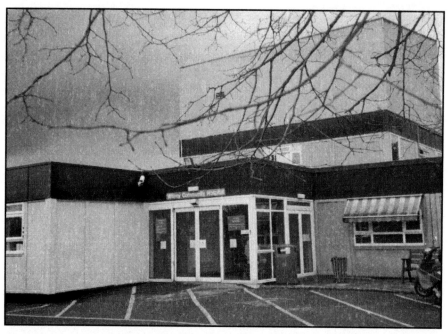

Witney Community Hospital.

my zimmer and took it again. It had fallen quite a lot.

At the same time the physio came from the discussion and said they had come to the conclusion that they should send me home where I might fare better. 'I have been in touch with your sister,' she said, 'It is all arranged.'

I was appalled. I couldn't stand, how could I possibly manage? My left leg was painful and I wasn't believed by anyone. There was no blame on Witney Hospital, they were doing their job. My operation scar had healed, I had a filter to prevent any clots getting to my heart. I should be oozing with energy... but I wasn't.

That same day Bridget was with me when I said my leg was worse; suddenly it had swollen right up to the groin, and I couldn't lift it off the bed.

She fetched Liz who was amazed, and put in motion a complete reversal of my routine. She called Dr. Sally who came and gave me four injections of warfarin. She looked at me and said, 'I'm very sorry Dorothy but I'll have to send you back to the J.R.'

12 A night on the tiles

They knew now what both Bridget and I had known weeks before, at the time when I wasn't listened to.

A blood clot had remained and now it was anchored and it would be there for ever. Did they or did they not know of its existence?

At the time when I left the J.R. originally I could not be treated with warfarin because of my operation scar. At the top of my drugs list was warfarin, starting date to be announced.

Now, with my left leg resembling a gatepost, and just as unyielding, I was transferred back to the J.R.

When entering the J.R. I was automatically placed on level six. This is the medical assessment unit. I was interviewed by a doctor during the night to ascertain the correct ward for me.

No one could possibly have imagined what I would encounter in that ward. I was put into a small portion of the ward meant, I think, for four beds, but there were already five in there and one place had been left for me in the corner.

A man was supposed to be next to me but he was insisting that he was not going to stay. He was stamping around the ward ripping down the curtains dressed only in his birthday suit. I had no idea that the curtains could be ripped down so easily or indeed re-hung so quickly.

Two males quickly tied the offender into his own bed and he carried on screaming.

'I am (and he shouted his name), but they call me Harry. I was born on February ** 192*, at least my head was, but they never told me when my feet were born. Jackie! Jackie! (not his wife's real name), come and get me. They have tied me up and left me outside the pub.'

That was his speech, we heard him shouting it as loudly as he could, over and over again. It was punctuated only by another man opposite whose plea was, 'Nurse, nurse, I want a pee.' If you remember a needle getting caught in an old record, that was the memory it brought back. I was extremely tired but it was a tiredness motivated by weakness.

This carried on for several hours, it didn't really worry me, I was quite amused by it. Another patient opposite me, who had 'Nil by mouth' over his bed, looked more disturbed by the situation.

Later that night a doctor came to see Harry and within seconds he had fallen asleep and slept for about twelve hours.

The doctor arrived at my bedside at 11:45pm. He remained until 1:00am. He discussed my left leg and I did tell him that I thought the clot was there even before I left the hospital the first time. I mentioned that Bridget had felt it, even saw it when my leg was silhouetted. 'I think your daughter was clever,' he said. 'It is very difficult to establish where clots are, in this case she was absolutely right.'

Even now I do not know why they didn't ask me about the pain. The pain from a blood clot is unlike any other pain I've ever had. Perhaps they knew and were balancing the worry of a haemorrhage and the chance of another clot.

He was very understanding, he explained everything to me, he confessed that there may be an improvement in my leg but it would never clear completely. He was very apologetic, he and I both knew that the filter had been inserted when it was a matter of life or death. This leg would make life more difficult but it was not life-threatening.

He explained the necessary details to me. First down to the X-ray unit, then on returning I was taken to the ultrascan unit. When I was shown the scan I could clearly see that the vein was now blocked to the groin.

I dozed intermittently all that day, and I must admit that as we patients were all so different, the food was not to the usual standard. I had had a bout of thrush so found it impossible to eat a sandwich. My daughters helped me out again.

I spent the day having injections and giving blood samples. I was not going to be transferred to another ward to avoid any risk of contacting that dreaded M.R.S.A.

I still had our friend 'Harry' in the next bed but he did not wake until nearly midday when his wife and his son came to visit. He was quite amiable now and conversed with us all including the nurses. He had had too many hours asleep, now he was wide awake, very energetic and in a good mood.

That gramophone needle was still caught in its groove opposite. Clearly the three of us plus three others were going to be there another night.

Harry sat up in bed in the evening, he was preparing us for another sleepless night.

'I'm nearly blind,' he said, 'But I can still sing.' That was true, his singing was beyond belief. He started with Irish songs, 'Mountains of Mourne', then 'Gypsy Rover', then 'Londonderry Air'. He followed on as if he had learned the sequence by heart.

Then he started on Scottish songs, 'Loch Lomond', 'Ye banks and Braes' and 'An Eriskay Love Lilt'. Then he started on English ones. He sang non-stop until he was given his midday meal the following day. That was probably about fourteen hours. Every word was pronounced clearly, every note was in tune and the production was straight.

Talking to Jackie in the morning, Harry was still singing. She said he had never had a music lesson, one of his parents came from Ireland and one from Scotland, but he had been brought up in England.

'Many landlords would ring him to ask for a musical evening. Remember you've only had that singing for one night, I've heard it for fifty years,' she said. I would love to meet him again, I will certainly never forget that night.

Going into hospital is like stepping into the unknown. You will meet a collection of human beings that have very little in common. It is up to each individual how you face the situation.

We all arrived here for one reason, namely that we needed help from the team of medical staff. We had a myriad of complaints caused by age, abuse of the body, hereditary background or even accidents. Cheerfulness between patients and nurses is the best way to overcome this situation.

After our midday meal both Harry and the patient opposite who was still stuck in his groove were transferred to other wards.

I was quite sad, I had enjoyed that singing, and I did not see Jackie again.

After about six days, the warfarin was monitored and I was returned to the community hospital at Witney.

13 Home again

I was welcomed back to Witney by friendly faces. I'd once again watch that corridor bounce, that commode run, that trolley serving knick-knacks controlled by women who give up their spare time to help. I'd see Joyce who – without fail – makes cups of tea every afternoon and visits each bed expecting no remuneration.

Such helpers work silently, all they want is a 'Thank you'.

There are many such helpers in all the hospitals I've been in. They sell in shops, run errands, arrange your flowers or even find their own jobs. These helpers are invaluable, they create a link between hospital and home.

One morning Sarah came in – that's the one with a ponytail – and offered a bath to the patient next to me, but the patient refused – she didn't need one, she blurted.

Now I heard all this and I had not had a bath lying down in hot water for years. I had made do with a shower because I couldn't get out of a bath. Was she refusing such a wholesome, beneficial, priceless commodity while I was being deprived? So I called Sarah and said 'Try me.' It was not within her powers to say 'yes' but she found Liz and was given the go-ahead.

I'll never forget that bath; a big thank you to Sarah! It was heavenly.

After a week or so my left leg started improving. I was not as quick returning to a normal life as I thought. My muscles had not been used for weeks so tiredness crept in very quickly. My left leg would not take my weight but I could progress with a zimmer.

One evening when Oxford United were playing at home, I asked Dr Sally if I could go. She agreed so, with the help of Liz, my son Colin decided to take me in a wheelchair. This was my first contact with the outside world. I enjoyed being in those same noisy surroundings that are so familiar to me. I forgot my own limitations for a while, but secretly I knew that I was not ready to enter that world quite yet. Thank you to all those who helped, I knew

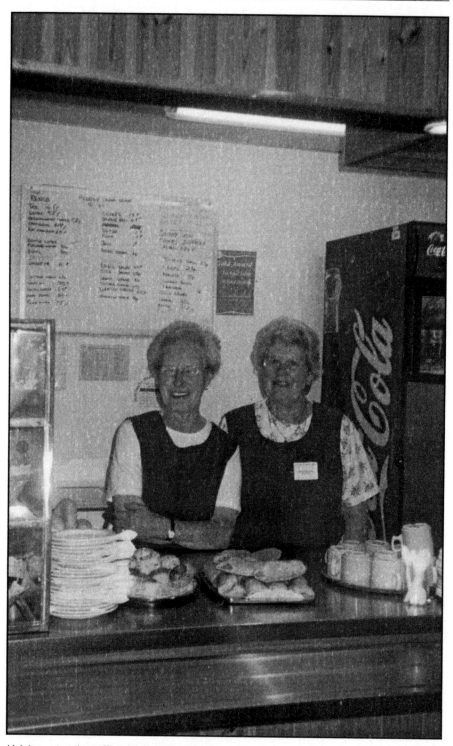

Helping out at the coffee shop.

that evening that one day I would be able to enter that hustle and bustle again.

It was a light at the end of the tunnel. Colin took me several times in a wheelchair and eventually with the zimmer.

Each day now I was improving but rather slowly because I'd been idle for a long time and even my good leg was very weak.

Eventually after more than one hundred days I was returning home. I had originally been told to expect to be in hospital for five days. The Noc could now cross one patient from their waiting list. I was in the J.R. much longer but they could not cross me off their list because I had never been on it.

On arriving home, I catered for myself. Living in a small village, I've always got a deep freeze full with plenty of choices.

After twenty-four hours at home the severe itching had disappeared. I was now convinced of the cause.

The physiotherapist came the following day, making sure I could get in and out of bed and could cook my meals. Things were very difficult, but I knew I had to do it. I've got a phone I carry with me if I manage to fall. I find a shower is very difficult and a bath impossible.

My daughter took me to the 'dialability centre' and they traced a dealer who would visit me and fit me with adjustable shoes.

Madge took me to whist drives, and if she could not manage it, another whist player would come and collect me. Colin made sure I didn't miss any football matches.

Any small jobs that I couldn't do would be done by anyone who called. My friend Mary collected my pension.

I would like to thank all the members of my family, parishioners of Combe and friends from far and wide who have helped me through this ordeal.

A special big thank you to Dr. Sally who helped far beyond the call of duty.

Don't forget the motto of this book. Read it, remember it and live by it. If you gave up smoking try spending your money on sport. Play it or watch it, it keeps you fit and helps bring nations closer together.

'I love Life'

This makes a good answer if you are tempted with an extra pint, a cigarette or even a second helping on your plate.

14 Looking forward with hope

I am now on the outside of the NHS again, looking in with a much broader knowledge.

This service is ours, not theirs. We are the ones who reap the benefit when we are in need.

I found each hospital very clean, each nurse very considerate. I was made to feel that I was the only one who occupied either their minds or their time. The meals were always good.

My own health was difficult, but I was never left to worry about any happenings. My hip replacement gave me no pain.

I did feel that an answer should have been found to the problem of the rash. That appeared to be unnecessary suffering.

My worst trouble was caused by haemorrhages. I received many packets of blood, but I did not feel selfish at using so much: both my husband and I had given freely in our younger days, when we both received a small red badge to be proud of. Thank you to all who are giving blood now: it is one of the best ways of helping our society.

Another way is to offer your organs at the end. I can't think that mine will be of any use, but as I won't be needing them again, why waste them?

It's nearly sixty years since we fought to get the NHS. Let's pull together and keep it in good health.

Postscript

When the heart stopped

When this happened to me I had never even thought about it and I don't think I would ever have known it had happened if my own doctor had not arrived at that exact moment.

I actually arrived at a beautiful place, the floor was mosaic but the texture was soft, it felt like soft rubber.

There was a strong, glowing light which engulfed the whole area.

The first person I met was Rose. She was a very great friend of mine who died quite suddenly a few years before.

'Oh, I am pleased to see you,' she said, 'but you must go back, it is not time for you yet.'

I wandered on and met my own father. He died in 1971.

'It's not time for you yet,' he said. He had a little boy with him. 'Is that my little boy?' I asked and he assured me that it was.

It was then that my doctor was saying 'Dorothy' and I opened my eyes to see her.

The check-up

I was called back to the Noc for a check up about six months later. They told me that my leg had very strong muscles which had caused the extensive operation scar.

I knew that my leg had very prominent muscles. I had always joked that my leg was more like a boxer's biceps than a female leg. Maybe it was caused by doing so much hard work for so many years.

When I asked why the clot in my left leg had not been detected when Bridget and I both knew it was there, the doctor – unlike the doctor at the J.R. – was most indignant, saying it was impossible for us to know. But hadn't we been proved right?

I hope that the origin of the rash will soon be sorted out. Apart from the irritation to the patient it would lessen the work of the nurses.

I think small improvements like these are the way forward.

ALSO BY DOROTHY CALCUTT

MY THREE HATS

The autobiography of a schoolgirl at Milham Ford, a member
of Stonesfield Silver Band, and a keen Oxford United supporter

This tale of personal adventure, triumph and tragedy, social change and rural
transformation, recalls the experiences of millions of country people strug-
gling to adapt to the rapid changes of the twentieth century.

£8 pbk   112 pages, illustrated

THE SALT OF THE EARTH

Diary of a poor family in Woodstock, 1900

One year in the life of a large family living on the edge of the Blenheim
Palace estate in Woodstock, Oxfordshire in 1900. The author's mother,
Dora, told her daughter many tales of her childhood at the turn of the
century, and this book is based on those stories. Includes contemporary
photographs of the people and places in the story.

£8 pbk   120pp

BORN IN A STABLE

The true story of John Ashton, illegitimate son of a
Northumberland nobleman and an Oxfordshire barmaid

Leo has inherited the family mansion in Northumberland, but is frustrated in
his desire to have a son to continue the name and inherit his estate. The
barmaid at an inn in the Oxfordshire village of Long Hanborough (Emma,
the author's great-grandmother) bears him a son, John. This book tells the
story of Leo's ambitions, of John's birth in extreme poverty in a farmyard
stable, and of his upbringing and occasional meetings with his father. The
events take place half a century before those in *The Salt of the Earth*.

£7.50 pbk   80pp

These books may be ordered post free from 01689 870437